I0503505

Hering's Law Applied to the Near Reflex

Louis S. Jagerman, MD

Hering's Law Applied to the Near Reflex

Louis S. Jagerman, MD
May 2014

Abstract

A study of 20 healthy young adults revealed that Hering's law operates in the pupillary and accommodative components of the near reflex. Dilatation or cycloplegia of one eye fixating at near instigates statistically significant excess miosis or excess accommodation in the other eye. These results revise conclusions reached with older methods and equipment.

Introduction

The near reflex is a binocular synkinesis of miosis, convergence, and accommodation of the eyes. This study, using modern methods and equipment, investigates whether Hering's law applies to the synergistic muscles entailed in the miosis and accommodation of the near reflex. The underlying concept is this: The naturally equal innervation of bilaterally symmetrical muscles guarantees that if one of these muscles is weakened so that excess effort is stimulated, the contralateral muscle will demonstrate excess contraction. In the case of eyes, a "weakening" can be achieved pharmacologically, as the sphincter of the pupil and the ciliary muscle of the uvea can be temporarily paralyzed with appropriate eye drops. The applicability of Hering's law to the innervation of the medial rectus muscles during natural convergence is already surmised. [1]

A pervious (1970) study on this issue indeed demonstrated excess miosis in a non-medicated near-fixating eye while the other "cyclopleged" eye fixates at near. [2] The same previous study also revealed excess accommodation under these conditions. However, dilatation without cycloplegia resulted in no significant miosis or accommodation in the contralateral eye. This study on just eight subjects used a simple pupil gauge (to the nearest ½ mm) and manual retinoscopy (to the nearest ¼ diopter) for detecting the pertinent changes through an oblique mirror, and computerized statistical analysis was in its infancy at that time.

The current (2014) study reconsiders these issues but goes further, using an objective automatic pupillometer, an automatic refractor, and modern computerized statistical software. Several benefits ensued: The use of hand-held monocular diagnostic devices simplified examining one eye while the other eye was fixating (e.g., no oblique mirror was needed). Pupillary size could be recorded to the nearest 1/10th mm. Mechanized refraction, set to 1/8th diopter steps, facilitated standardizing the retinoscopic technique. Finally, the large amount of data on 20 subjects could be analyzed digitally and could be readily subjected to more sophisticated analysis than was impossible 44 years earlier.

An additional issue was now addressed: Does mydriasis (dilatation) alone, without cycloplegia, actually elude Hering's law? That was the 1970 inference, since no statistically significant excess changes were found in miosis upon simply dilating the other pupil. Using a larger sample and more modern equipment and methods, is this conclusion valid?

Materials and Methods

Twenty (20) generally and ophthalmologically healthy subjects were accepted for their ability to hold fixation at distance or near with either eye while the contralateral eye was examined. Since this study only considered a normal physiological process, extraneous factors were excluded as much as possible. Thus very myopic, slightly hyperopic, slightly astigmatic, and all presbyopic individuals were excluded. For the same reason individuals with heterotropias, unusual heterophorias, abnormal binocular fusion, or significant anisometropia were disqualified. The ages ranged from 22 to 29 years and averaged 25.5, equally divided between men and women. All were right-eye dominant. No consideration was given to iris color or race.

The equipment included A Welch-Allyn (Skaneateles Falls, NY 13152 USA) SureSight ® hand-held autorefractor set for adults and for $1/8^{th}$ diopter steps. An MPI™-100 NeurOptics (Ivine, CA 92612 USA) hand-held Pupillometer was used to measure the initial instant pupil size to the nearest $1/10^{th}$ mm. The data were organized and analyzed on a MacBook Pro computer with MS Excel. (Apple ® OS X version 10.7.5; Microsoft Excel ® for Mac 2011 version 14.2.0.)

The medications were Phenylephrine HCl 10% (Akorn Pharmaceuticals, Decatur, Ill 62522) and Cyclogyl 2% (Alcon Laboratories, Fort Worth Tx, 76134). These are familiar commercially available preparations routinely used in clinical ocular examination and in various therapeutic settings. The author and his assistants have no financial interest in any of the manufacturers.

Several precautions were taken: Only fresh medications were administered, these were refrigerated, and they were used exclusively for this study. Two drops of each medication were given. A half hour after Phenylephrine and one hour after Cyclogyl was allowed to elapse before any measurement was begun. Enough delay was allowed between examinations to let drug effects wear off completely; hence the study took about eight weeks. No other eye drops were allowed. None of the subjects was on any systemic or topical medication. Health changes were closely monitored; indeed none were reported, and none of the 20 subjects became ill during the study, so that no alternates had to be called in. All testing was done in the same room, and a constant lighting level was maintained, including of course when pupillary sizes were measured. Care was taken to randomize which eye was studied first. One examiner, the author, performed all experimental measurements.

Several definitions used in this study should be spelled out:

"Sphere" is the spherical-equivalent refraction. (Please note that the selection of subjects favored small refractive errors and allowed only negligible astigmatism.)

"Distance Rx" is the refraction of the examined eye while the contralateral fixates at 6 meters.

"Near Rx" is the refraction of the examined eye while the contralateral eye fixates at 20 cm (1/5th of one meter).

"Dilated" means medicated with only Phenylephrine. I.e., mydriasis without cycloplegia was induced. (Of course cycloplegia is accompanied by dilatation.)

"Cyclopleged" (admittedly not a recognized English verb) means medicated with Cyclogyl. I.e., cycloplegia was induced, of course along with mydriasis.

"Accommodation" means the algebraic difference between the near and distance refractions, with or without medication, even when the two measurements are obtained at different occasions.

"Excess miosis" is the algebraic difference in the amount of pupil construction without medication vs. with medication in the other eye, be it for dilatation or cycloplegia. The goal of the study was to elicit excess miosis under the experimental conditions.

"Excess accommodation" is the algebraic difference in the amount of accommodation without medication vs. with medication in the other eye, be it for dilatation or cycloplegia. The goal of the study was also to elicit excess accommodation under the experimental conditions.

"Refraction" with the Welch-Allyn refractor was not done in the standard manner, wherein the patient should fixate a target inside the device. Rather, one eye was refracted while the other fixated elsewhere, specifically at 6 meters or 20 cm. [3, 4] (The selection of subjects favored persons capable of cooperating in this manner, and none reported any difficulty.)

The "size" of the pupils was measured with the NeurOptics Pupillometer; only the initial instant minimal size was recorded, before any hippus could occur. [5] (This pupillometer also tracks the pupil size for several seconds after the initial measurement, as is useful in neurologic assessment, but this function was irrelevant here.)

Statistical analyses were done on the two eyes of each subject separately, lest the natural interdependence of the pair skew the results. Thus eight experimental conditions were analyzed. Four of these were aimed at detecting excess accommodation, and the other four were aimed at detecting excess miosis, though null hypotheses were applied in the analyses. Here are these eight conditions:

Accommodation of right eyes without medication vs. their accommodation while dilated.

Accommodation of left eyes without medication vs. their accommodation while dilated.

Accommodation of right eyes without medication vs. their accommodation while cyclopeged.

Accommodation of left eyes without medication vs. their accommodation while cyclopleged.

Miosis of right eyes without medication vs. their miosis while dilated.

Miosis of left eyes without medication vs. their miosis while dilated.

Miosis of right eyes without medication vs. their miosis while cyclopeged.

Miosis of left eyes without medication vs. their miosis while cyclopleged.

Results

In all eight experimental conditions, the following results were statistically significant: *Excess miosis or excess accommodation was evident in the contralateral eyes when the fixating pupil was dilated or when the fixating eye was cyclopleged.*

These results are interpreted further under "discussion," but apparently when a pupil—for example the right—is dilated while the right eye fixates at near, the left eye receives enough nerve stimulation to over-constrict the left pupil. That is to say, the left pupil becomes smaller than it would have been if the right eye were not medicated with a mydriatic. Thus the left pupil exhibits excess miosis.

Similarly, when an eye—again for instance the right—is cyclopeged while the right eye fixates at near, the left eye receives enough nerve stimulation to over-accommodate. That is to say, the left ciliary body muscle overacts compared with its action if the right eye were not medicated with a cycloplegic. Thus the left eye exhibits excess accommodation.

Although right and left eyes were analyzed separately, and although right-left differences were encountered (amounts of accommodation and miosis were not always symmetric), none of the right-left discrepancies altered the statistical significance of the principal findings.

The following table (Table 1) shows the key numeric values. For simplicity, data from right and left eyes are pooled, and each value is a mean (average).

	Dilated	Cyclopleged
Excess miosis (millimeters)	0.43	1.08
Excess accommodation (diopters)	1.23	3.02

Table 1. Summary of principal results.

For clarity in interpreting the above table, here is a review of the "Excess miosis, Dilated" case as an example: The size of the pupil had been measured without medication while fixating at 20 cm., and this datum represents the natural miosis of the near reflex. One eye was then medicated to dilate its pupil and then made to fixate at 20 cm. while the size of the other pupil was measured. On average, the size of this "other" non-medicated eye was found to be 0.43 millimeters smaller than the "natural" miosis detected at 20 cm. when neither eye had been medicated. This difference was recorded as the excess miosis under the experimental condition; i.e., an additional 0.43 millimeters of miosis was elicited.

The same concepts govern the cases wherein accommodation was considered, except of course refractions were performed to obtain the amount of natural accommodation of the near reflex and later to obtain the amount of excess (additional) accommodation while the fixating eye was cyclopeged. Of course the unit of accommodation is the diopter.

Another set of results was obtained "behind the scenes." These data are not directly pertinent to the above principal results but they served auxiliary purposes. They are only summarized in this publication, as the details would require several pages, but they are available on request (in the form of a Microsoft Excel ® file containing a large spread sheet).

In particular, the distance and rear refractions without medication were recorded for each subject. This information allowed the calculation (by subtraction) of the amount of natural accommodation for each subject. The mean of the subjects' distance refraction was −1.50 diopters (spherical equivalent) and the mean near Rx was −6.039. Ergo, the mean accommodation for 20 cm. was 4.539 diopters. This agrees closely with optical theory (5 diopters) and with other studies. [6] All subjects showed this kind of refractive reaction to fixation at near. (Clinical refraction to 1/1000th of a diopter is impossible, but these values are useful in the statistics.)

Although this information was not used in calculations (direct measurements sufficed), the mean of the pupil size at distance was found to be 5.35 mm and at near was 2.90, suggesting that the natural near reflex was accompanied by 2.45 mm of miosis in the conditions of this study. This also agrees with past experience, [7] and it confirms that every subject showed the expected pupillary reaction to fixation at near in the absence of medications.

The statistical calculations, using standard and familiar equations, are summarized as follows. As is customary, null hypotheses were presumed, namely that neither medication would provoke excess pupillary changes or excess refractive changes. For example, a null hypothesis would posit that the mean accommodation at near without medication (4.574 diopters) was not significantly different from the accommodation while the other eye was dilated (5.792 diopters).

Eight mean-to-mean comparisons (as listed above) were subjected to analysis, using Student's t-test at the 0.05 confidence level. In any of these cases a null hypothesis could be rejected with 95% confidence if the calculated t-value exceeded the critical t-value. (One set of t-values evaluates a pair of means.) As shown in table 2, the null hypothesis could be rejected in all eight cases; that is to say, in each case mathematical a comparison of the two appropriate means indicated a statistically significant difference between them.

Modern software-based applications of Student's test also include presentation of a p-value for each comparison, which expresses the likelihood that the null hypothesis was erroneously rejected; the smaller this value, the more strongly the data justify this rejection. (One p-value evaluates a pair of means.) All eight p-values were sufficiently small to conclude that in each case a statistically significant excess effect had occurred.

Analysis of each mean provided two additional statistical values: a standard deviation (a measure of the scatter of the 20 values that had been averaged), and a standard error (the standard deviation divided by $\sqrt{20}$, hence a measure of scatter considering the sample size.) These results suggest that the measurements on these subjects (all carefully selected) did not exhibit objectionable variances.

The next table presents these results, to a level of precision that could not be achieved in the study of 1970.

Experimental condition		Statistical data			
		Without medication	With medication		
Accommodation OD without medication vs. dilated.	Mean	4.574	5.792	Calculated t	8.373
	S. D.	0.3521	0.5471	Critical t	1.686
	S. E.	0.0787	0.1223	P-value	3.72
Accommodation OS without medication vs. dilated.	Mean	4.505	5.749	Calculated t	4.996
	S. D.	0.641	0.911	Critical t	1.686
	S. E.	0.1433	0.2036	P-value	1.35
Accommodation OD without medication vs. cyclopleged.	Mean	4.574	7.612	Calculated t	21.748
	S. D.	0.3521	0.516	Critical t	1.686
	S. E.	0.0787	0.1154	P-value	4.80
Accommodation OS without medication vs. cyclopleged.	Mean	4.505	7.506	Calculated t	14.140
	S. D.	0.641	0.670	Critical t	1.686
	S. E.	0.1433	0.1565	P-value	1.02
Miosis OD without medication vs. dilated.	Mean	2.91	2.46	Calculated t	3.921
	S. D.	0.3892	0.3347	Critical t	1.686
	S. E.	0.087	0.0745	P-value	0.0004
Miosis OS without medication vs. dilated.	Mean	2.89	2.49	Calculated t	3.201
	S. D.	0.3959	0.4042	Critical t	1.686
	S. E.	0.0885	0.0904	P-value	0.003
Miosis OD without medication vs. cyclopleged.	Mean	2.91	1.83	Calculated t	10.277
	S. D.	0.3892	0.2673	Critical t	1.686
	S. E.	0.087	0.0598	P-value	1.59
Miosis OS without medication vs. cycloplged.	Mean	2.89	1.83	Calculated t	10.112
	S. D.	0.3959	0.2552	Critical t	1.686
	S. E.	0.0885	0.5707	P-value	2.51

Table 2. Statistical values for the eight experimental conditions.

For interested readers in the mathematics, the tables on the next 8 pages show the statistical calculations in the same order as the above 8 possible experimental conditions. Each page in effect is an individual application of the Student's t-test and shows the raw data.

Pages 19 and 20 show the autorefractor and the pupillometer used in the study.

ACCOMMODATION OD WITHOUT MEDICATION VS. DILATED

	INDIVIDUAL	SAMPLES - GROUPS - TREATMENT GROUPS				
		SAMPLE 1		SAMPLE 2		
		$X_{i,1}$	$X_{i,1}^2$	$X_{i,2}$	$X_{i,2}^2$	Use this test to compare two samples (groups, treatments) for a significant difference. Goal is the computed t ratio. Numerator will be the difference between the two sample means. Denominator will be the standard deviation of the difference between these means. Difference apt to be significant if small st. dev. of diff. bet. means and large sample sizes.
	1	4.87	23.7169	5.50	30.25	
	2	4.12	16.9744	5.50	30.25	
	3	4.00	16	5.75	33.0625	
	4	4.75	22.5625	4.87	23.7169	
	5	4.88	23.8144	5.25	27.5625	
	6	4.50	20.25	5.37	28.8369	
	7	4.63	21.4369	5.63	31.6969	
	8	4.62	21.3444	5.00	25	
	9	4.50	20.25	5.12	26.2144	
	10	4.75	22.5625	5.87	34.4569	
	11	4.50	20.25	6.37	40.5769	
	12	4.00	16	5.37	28.8369	
	13	4.87	23.7169	6.12	37.4544	
	14	4.75	22.5625	6.50	42.25	
	15	4.87	23.7169	6.75	45.5625	
	16	3.88	15.0544	6.00	36	
	17	5.13	26.3169	6.63	43.9569	
	18	4.50	20.25	6.00	36	
	19	5.00	25	6.25	39.0625	
	20	4.37	19.0969	6.00	36	
Size of sample n		20		20		Need NOT be same
Sum $X_i = \Sigma x_i = \Sigma x$		91.49		115.85		Sum of x's
Sample means $(\Sigma x_i)/n = \bar{x}$		4.5745		5.7925		The difference between these means will be the numerator of t ratio. (Absolute value.)
Sum of Squares $\Sigma(X_i)^2 = \Sigma x^2$			420.8765		676.7471	Sums of Squares
Square of sum $(\Sigma X_i)^2 = (\Sigma x)^2$		8370.4		13421.2		Squares of sums
$\dfrac{(\Sigma x)^2}{n}$		418.52		671.061		"Grand mean" Also used in ANOVA
Σd^2		2.3555		5.68601		$\Sigma d^2 = \Sigma x^2 - \dfrac{(\Sigma x)^2}{n}$ "SS$_T$"
Variances σ_1^2 and σ_2^2	Note one variance for EACH MEAN	0.124		0.29926		$\sigma^2 = \Sigma d^2 / (n-1) = $ Variance.
σ_d^2		0.0212				$\sigma_d^2 = \dfrac{\sigma_1^2}{n_1} + \dfrac{\sigma_2^2}{n_2}$ "Pooled" variance of difference between
σ_d	Note ONE standard deviation.	0.1455				Square root of variance σ_d^2. Standard deviation of difference between means. Denominator.
$t_{computed}$		-8.3728	Ignore sign if negative. (Absolute value.)			$t = \dfrac{\bar{X}_1 - \bar{X}_2}{\sigma_d}$ The t ratio. Computed t.
df		19		19		Degrees of freedom. Each df = n - 1.
We have total of		38 degrees of freedom all together.				

Table t for p=0.05 & 0.01 = 1.686 & 2.429. Since computed t is larger, **reject null hypothesis.**

ACCOMMODATION OS WITHOUT MEDICATION VS. DILATED

SAMPLES - GROUPS - TREATMENT GROUPS

INDIVIDUAL	SAMPLE 1 $X_{i,1}$	$X_{i,1}^2$	SAMPLE 2 $X_{i,2}$	$X_{i,2}^2$
1	4.87	23.7169	5.62	31.5844
2	3.87	14.9769	5.25	27.5625
3	4.00	16	6.00	36
4	5.12	26.2144	5.00	25
5	4.50	20.25	4.87	23.7169
6	4.50	20.25	5.25	27.5625
7	4.25	18.0625	5.25	27.5625
8	3.12	9.7344	3.50	12.25
9	4.25	18.0625	4.87	23.7169
10	4.25	18.0625	5.62	31.5844
11	4.50	20.25	6.50	42.25
12	3.75	14.0625	5.12	26.2144
13	4.87	23.7169	6.00	36
14	3.88	15.0544	5.63	31.6969
15	4.87	23.7169	6.75	45.5625
16	4.25	18.0625	6.37	40.5769
17	5.50	30.25	7.25	52.5625
18	5.00	25	6.25	39.0625
19	5.87	34.4569	7.00	49
20	4.87	23.7169	6.87	47.1969

Use this test to compare two samples (groups, treatments) for a significant difference. Goal is the computed t ratio. Numerator will be the difference between the two sample means. Denominator will be the standard deviation of the difference between these means. Difference apt to be significant if small st. dev. of diff. bet. means and large sample sizes.

	Sample 1	Sample 2	
Size of sample n	20	20	Need NOT be same.
Sum $X_i = \Sigma x_i = \Sigma x$	90.09	114.97	Sum of x's
Sample means $(\Sigma x_i)/n = \bar{x}$	4.5045	5.7485	The difference between these means will be the numerator of t ratio. (Absolute value.)
Sum of Squares $\Sigma(X_i)^2 = \Sigma x^2$	413.6171	676.6627	Sums of Squares
Square of sum $(\Sigma X_i)^2 = (\Sigma x)^2$	8116.2	13218.1	Squares of sums
$\frac{(\Sigma x)^2}{n}$	405.81	660.905	"Grand mean" — Also used in ANOVA
Σd^2	7.8067	15.7577	$\Sigma d^2 = \Sigma x^2 - \frac{(\Sigma x)^2}{n}$ "SS$_T$"
Variances σ_1^2 and σ_2^2 (Note one variance for EACH MEAN)	0.4109	0.82935	$\sigma^2 = \Sigma d^2 / (n-1) = $ Variance.
σ_d^2	0.062		$\sigma_d^2 = \frac{\sigma_1^2}{n_1} + \frac{\sigma_2^2}{n_2}$ "Pooled" variance of difference between
σ_d (Note ONE standard deviation.)	0.249		Square root of variance σ_d^2. Standard deviation of difference between means. Denominator.
$t_{computed}$	-4.9956 (Ignore sign if negative. (Absolute value.))		$t = \frac{\bar{X}_1 - \bar{X}_2}{\sigma_d}$ The t ratio. Computed t.
df	19	19	Degrees of freedom. Each df = n - 1.

We have total of 38 degrees of freedom all together.

Table t for p=0.05 & 0.01 = 1.686 & 2.429. Since computed t is larger, **reject null hypothesis.**

9

ACOMMODATION OD WITHOUT MEDICATION VS. CYCLOPLEGED

SAMPLES - GROUPS - TREATMENT GROUPS

INDIVIDUAL	SAMPLE 1 $X_{i,1}$	$X_{i,1}^2$	SAMPLE 2 $X_{i,2}$	$X_{i,2}^2$	
1	4.87	23.7169	6.50	42.25	Use this test to compare two samples (groups, treatments) for a significant difference. Goal is the computed t ratio. Numerator will be the difference between the two sample means. Denominator will be the standard deviation of the difference between these means. Difference apt to be significant if small st. dev. of diff. bet. means and large sample sizes.
2	4.12	16.9744	7.37	54.3169	
3	4.00	16	6.75	45.5625	
4	4.75	22.5625	7.25	52.5625	
5	4.88	23.8144	7.63	58.2169	
6	4.50	20.25	7.00	49	
7	4.63	21.4369	7.63	58.2169	
8	4.62	21.3444	7.62	58.0644	
9	4.50	20.25	8.25	68.0625	
10	4.75	22.5625	7.25	52.5625	
11	4.50	20.25	7.50	56.25	
12	4.00	16	8.37	70.0569	
13	4.87	23.7169	7.75	60.0625	
14	4.75	22.5625	7.87	61.9369	
15	4.87	23.7169	8.00	64	
16	3.88	15.0544	8.13	66.0969	
17	5.13	26.3169	8.50	72.25	
18	4.50	20.25	7.50	56.25	
19	5.00	25	7.88	62.0944	
20	4.37	19.0969	7.50	56.25	

Size of sample n		20	20	Need NOT be same	
Sum $X_i = \Sigma x_i = \Sigma x$		91.49	152.25	Sum of x's	
Sample means $(\Sigma x_i)/n = \bar{x}$		4.5745	7.6125	The difference between these means will be the numerator of t ratio. (Absolute value.)	
Sum of Squares $\Sigma(X_i)^2 = \Sigma x^2$		420.8765	1164.063	Sums of Squares	
Square of sum $(\Sigma X_i)^2 = (\Sigma x)^2$		8370.4	23180.1	Squares of sums	
$\frac{(\Sigma x)^2}{n}$		418.52	1159	"Grand mean"	Also used in ANOVA
Σd^2		2.3555	5.05963	$\Sigma d^2 = \Sigma x^2 - \frac{(\Sigma x)^2}{n}$	"SS$_T$"
Variances σ_1^2 and σ_2^2	Note one variance for EACH MEAN	0.124	0.2663	$\sigma^2 = \Sigma d^2 / (n-1) = $ Variance.	
σ_d^2		0.0195		$\sigma_d^2 = \frac{\sigma_1^2}{n_1} + \frac{\sigma_2^2}{n_2}$	"Pooled" variance of difference between
σ_d	Note ONE standard deviation.	0.1397		Square root of variance σ_d^2. Standard deviation of difference between means. Denominator.	
$t_{computed}$		-21.748	Ignore sign if negative. (Absolute value.)	$t = \frac{\bar{X}_1 - \bar{X}_2}{\sigma_d}$	The t ratio. Computed t.
df		19	19	Degrees of freedom. Each df = n - 1.	
We have total of		38	degrees of freedom all together.		

Table t for p=0.05 & 0.01 = 1.686 & 2.429. Since computed t is larger, **reject null hypothesis.**

ACCOMMODATION OS WITHOUT MEDICATION VS. CYCLOPLEGED

SAMPLES - GROUPS - TREATMENT GROUPS

INDIVIDUAL	SAMPLE 1 $X_{i,1}$	$X_{i,1}^2$	SAMPLE 2 $X_{i,2}$	$X_{i,2}^2$	
1	4.87	23.7169	6.87	47.1969	Use this test to compare two samples (groups, treatments) for a significant difference. Goal is the computed t ratio. Numerator will be the difference between the two sample means. Denominator will be the standard deviation of the difference between these means. Difference apt to be significant if small st. dev. of diff. bet. means and large sample sizes.
2	3.87	14.9769	7.00	49	
3	4.00	16	6.75	45.5625	
4	5.12	26.2144	7.50	56.25	
5	4.50	20.25	7.00	49	
6	4.50	20.25	7.00	49	
7	4.25	18.0625	7.50	56.25	
8	3.12	9.7344	6.00	36	
9	4.25	18.0625	8.00	64	
10	4.25	18.0625	7.00	49	
11	4.50	20.25	7.62	58.0644	
12	3.75	14.0625	8.00	64	
13	4.87	23.7169	8.12	65.9344	
14	3.88	15.0544	7.13	50.8369	
15	4.87	23.7169	8.50	72.25	
16	4.25	18.0625	7.25	52.5625	
17	5.50	30.25	8.87	78.6769	
18	5.00	25	7.75	60.0625	
19	5.87	34.4569	8.50	72.25	
20	4.87	23.7169	7.75	60.0625	

Size of sample n		20		20	Need NOT be same
Sum $X_i = \Sigma x_i = \Sigma x$		90.09		150.11	Sum of x's
Sample means $(\Sigma x_i)/n = \bar{x}$		4.5045		7.5055	The difference between these means will be the numerator of t ratio. (Absolute value.)
Sum of Squares $\Sigma(X_i)^2 = \Sigma x^2$			413.6171		1135.96	Sums of Squares
Square of sum $(\Sigma X_i)^2 = (\Sigma x)^2$		8116.2		22533	Squares of sums
$\dfrac{(\Sigma x)^2}{n}$		405.81		1126.65	"Grand mean" — Also used in ANOVA
Σd^2		7.8067		9.30895	$\Sigma d^2 = \Sigma x^2 - \dfrac{(\Sigma x)^2}{n}$ — "SS$_T$"
Variances σ_1^2 and σ_2^2	Note one variance for EACH MEAN	0.4109		0.48994	$\sigma^2 = \Sigma d^2 / (n-1) = $ Variance.
σ_d^2		0.045			$\sigma_d^2 = \dfrac{\sigma_1^2}{n_1} + \dfrac{\sigma_2^2}{n_2}$ — "Pooled" variance of difference between
σ_d	Note ONE standard deviation.	0.2122			Square root of variance σ_d^2. Standard deviation of difference between means. Denominator.
$t_{computed}$		-14.14	Ignore sign if negative. (Absolute value.)		$t = \left\lvert \dfrac{\bar{X}_1 - \bar{X}_2}{\sigma_d} \right\rvert$ — The t ratio. Computed t.
df		19		19	Degrees of freedom. Each df = n - 1.

We have total of **38** degrees of freedom all together.

Table t for p=0.05 & 0.01 = 1.686 & 2.429. Since computed t is larger, **reject null hypothesis.**

MIOSIS OD WITHOUT MEDICATION VS. DILATED

	INDIVIDUAL	SAMPLE 1		SAMPLE 2		
SAMPLES - GROUPS - TREATMENT GROUPS		$X_{i,1}$	$X_{i,1}^2$	$X_{i,2}$	$X_{i,2}^2$	
	1	3.1	9.61	2.5	6.25	Use this test to compare two samples (groups, treatments) for a significant difference. Goal is the computed t ratio. Numerator will be the difference between the two sample means. Denominator will be the standard deviation of the difference between these means. Difference apt to be significant if small st. dev. of diff. bet. means and large sample sizes.
	2	3.7	13.69	3.0	9	
	3	3.6	12.96	2.5	6.25	
	4	2.7	7.29	2.5	6.25	
	5	3.0	9	2.5	6.25	
	6	3.0	9	2.5	6.25	
	7	2.4	5.76	2.1	4.41	
	8	2.6	6.76	2.4	5.76	
	9	2.8	7.84	2.0	4	
	10	2.9	8.41	2.1	4.41	
	11	2.6	6.76	2.5	6.25	
	12	3.0	9	2.6	6.76	
	13	2.3	5.29	2.2	4.84	
	14	2.8	7.84	2.0	4	
	15	2.4	5.76	2.1	4.41	
	16	2.6	6.76	2.3	5.29	
	17	2.8	7.84	2.5	6.25	
	18	3.3	10.89	3.0	9	
	19	3.3	10.89	3.2	10.24	
	20	3.3	10.89	2.7	7.29	
Size of sample n		20		20		Need NOT be same
Sum $X_i = \Sigma x_i = \Sigma x$		58.2		49.2		Sum of x's
Sample means $(\Sigma x_i)/n = \bar{x}$		2.91		2.46		The difference between these means will be the numerator of t ratio. (Absolute value.)
Sum of Squares $\Sigma(X_i)^2 = \Sigma x^2$			172.24		123.16	Sums of Squares
Square of sum $(\Sigma X_i)^2 = (\Sigma x)^2$		3387.2		2420.64		Squares of sums
$\frac{(\Sigma x)^2}{n}$		169.36		121.032		"Grand mean" Also used in ANOVA
Σd^2		2.878		2.12801		$\Sigma d^2 = \Sigma x^2 - \frac{(\Sigma x)^2}{n}$ "SS$_T$"
Variances σ_1^2 and σ_2^2	Note one variance for EACH MEAN	0.1515		0.112		$\sigma^2 = \Sigma d^2 / (n-1)$ = Variance.
σ_d^2		0.0132				$\sigma_d^2 = \frac{\sigma_1^2}{n_1} + \frac{\sigma_2^2}{n_2}$ "Pooled" variance of difference between
σ_d	Note ONE standard deviation.	0.1148				Square root of variance σ_d^2. Standard deviation of difference between means. Denominator.
$t_{computed}$		3.9207	Ignore sign if negative. (Absolute value.)			$t = \dfrac{\bar{X}_1 - \bar{X}_2}{\sigma_d}$ The t ratio. Computed t.
df		19		19		Degrees of freedom. Each df = n - 1.
We have total of		38 degrees of freedom all together.				

Table t for p=0.05 & 0.01 = 1.686 & 2.429. Since computed t is larger, **reject null hypothesis.**

MIOSIS OS WITHOUT MEDICATION VS. DILATED

	INDIVIDUAL	SAMPLE 1		SAMPLE 2		SAMPLES - GROUPS - TREATMENT GROUPS	
		$X_{i,1}$	$X_{i,1}^2$	$X_{i,2}$	$X_{i,2}^2$		
	1	3.1	9.61	2.0	4	Use this test to compare two samples (groups, treatments) for a significant difference. Goal is the computed t ratio. Numerator will be the difference between the two sample means. Denominator will be the standard deviation of the difference between these means. Difference apt to be significant if small st. dev. of diff. bet. means and large sample sizes.	
	2	3.7	13.69	2.5	6.25		
	3	3.6	12.96	2.5	6.25		
	4	2.7	7.29	2.5	6.25		
	5	2.9	8.41	3.0	9		
	6	3.0	9	2.5	6.25		
	7	2.3	5.29	2.1	4.41		
	8	2.6	6.76	2.4	5.76		
	9	2.8	7.84	2.1	4.41		
	10	3.0	9	2.1	4.41		
	11	2.5	6.25	2.5	6.25		
	12	2.9	8.41	2.4	5.76		
	13	2.3	5.29	2.2	4.84		
	14	2.8	7.84	1.9	3.61		
	15	2.4	5.76	2.2	4.84		
	16	2.6	6.76	3.4	11.56		
	17	2.8	7.84	2.5	6.25		
	18	3.3	10.89	3.1	9.61		
	19	3.2	10.24	3.1	9.61		
	20	3.3	10.89	2.7	7.29		

Size of sample n		20		20	NEED NOT be same
Sum $X_i = \Sigma x_i = \Sigma x$		57.8		49.7	Sum of x's
Sample means $(\Sigma x_i)/n = \bar{x}$		2.89		2.485	The difference between these means will be the numerator of t ratio. (Absolute value.)
Sum of Squares $\Sigma(X_i)^2 = \Sigma x^2$			170.02	126.61	Sums of Squares
Square of sum $(\Sigma X_i)^2 = (\Sigma x)^2$		3340.8		2470.09	Squares of sums
$\dfrac{(\Sigma x)^2}{n}$		167.04		123.504	"Grand mean" Also used in ANOVA
Σd^2		2.978		3.10551	$\Sigma_d^2 = \Sigma_x^2 - \dfrac{(\Sigma x)^2}{n}$ "SS$_T$"
Variances σ_1^2 and σ_2^2	Note one variance for EACH MEAN	0.1567		0.16345	$\sigma^2 = \Sigma d^2 / (n-1) = $ Variance.
σ_d^2		0.016			$\sigma_d^2 = \dfrac{\sigma_1^2}{n_1} + \dfrac{\sigma_2^2}{n_2}$ "Pooled" variance of difference between
σ_d	Note ONE standard deviation.	0.1265			Square root of variance σ_d^2. Standard deviation of difference between means. Denominator.
$t_{computed}$		3.2009	Ignore sign if negative. (Absolute value.)		$t = \dfrac{\bar{X}_1 - \bar{X}_2}{\sigma_d}$ The t ratio. Computed t.
df		19		19	Degrees of freedom. Each df = n - 1.

We have total of **38** degrees of freedom all together.

Table t for p=0.05 & 0.01 = 1.686 & 2.429. Since computed t is larger, **reject null hypothesis.**

MIOSIS OD WITHOUT MEDICATION VS. CYCLOPLEGED

SAMPLES - GROUPS - TREATMENT GROUPS

	INDIVIDUAL	SAMPLE 1		SAMPLE 2			Use this test to compare two samples (groups, treatments) for a significant difference. Goal is the computed t ratio. Numerator will be the difference between the two sample means. Denominator will be the standard deviation of the difference between these means. Difference apt to be significant if small st. dev. of diff. bet. means and large sample sizes.
		$X_{i,1}$	$X_{i,1}^2$	$X_{i,2}$	$X_{i,2}^2$		
	1	3.1	9.61	1.5	2.25		
	2	3.7	13.69	1.6	2.56		
	3	3.6	12.96	2.3	5.29		
	4	2.7	7.29	1.7	2.89		
	5	3.0	9	2.0	4		
	6	3.0	9	1.8	3.24		
	7	2.4	5.76	2.0	4		
	8	2.6	6.76	1.5	2.25		
	9	2.8	7.84	2.0	4		
	10	2.9	8.41	2.1	4.41		
	11	2.6	6.76	2.2	4.84		
	12	3.0	9	1.5	2.25		
	13	2.3	5.29	1.6	2.56		
	14	2.8	7.84	1.7	2.89		
	15	2.4	5.76	1.4	1.96		
	16	2.6	6.76	1.6	2.56		
	17	2.8	7.84	2.0	4		
	18	3.3	10.89	2.1	4.41		
	19	3.3	10.89	1.9	3.61		
	20	3.3	10.89	2.0	4		
Size of sample n		20		20		Need NOT be same	
Sum $X_i = \Sigma x_i = \Sigma x$		58.2		36.5		Sum of x's	
Sample means $(\Sigma x_i)/n = \bar{x}$		2.91		1.825		The difference between these means will be the numerator of t ratio. (Absolute value.)	
Sum of Squares $\Sigma(X_i)^2 = \Sigma x^2$			172.24		67.97	Sums of Squares	
Square of sum $(\Sigma X_i)^2 = (\Sigma x)^2$		3387.2		1332.25		Squares of sums	
$\dfrac{(\Sigma x)^2}{n}$		169.36		66.6125		"Grand mean"	Also used in ANOVA
Σd^2		2.878		1.3575		$\Sigma d^2 = \Sigma x^2 - \dfrac{(\Sigma x)^2}{n}$	"SS$_T$"
Variances σ_1^2 and σ_2^2	Note one variance for EACH MEAN	0.1515		0.07145		$\sigma^2 = \Sigma d^2 / (n-1) = $ Variance.	
σ_d^2		0.0111				$\sigma_d^2 = \dfrac{\sigma_1^2}{n_1} + \dfrac{\sigma_2^2}{n_2}$	"Pooled" variance of difference between
σ_d	Note ONE standard deviation.	0.1056				Square root of variance σ_d^2. Standard deviation of difference between means. Denominator.	
$t_{computed}$		10.277	Ignore sign if negative. (Absolute value.)			$t = \dfrac{\bar{x}_1 - \bar{x}_2}{\sigma_d}$	The t ratio. Computed t.
df		19		19		Degrees of freedom. Each df = n - 1.	
We have total of		38	degrees of freedom all together.				

Table t for p=0.05 & 0.01 = 1.686 & 2.429. Since computed t is larger, **reject null hypothesis.**

MIOSIS OS WITHOUT MEDICATION VS. CYCLOPLEGED

SAMPLES - GROUPS - TREATMENT GROUPS

INDIVIDUAL	SAMPLE 1		SAMPLE 2		
	$X_{i,1}$	$X_{i,1}^2$	$X_{i,2}$	$X_{i,2}^2$	Use this test to compare two samples (groups, treatments) for a significant difference. Goal is the computed t ratio. Numerator will be the difference between the two sample means. Denominator will be the standard deviation of the difference between these means. Difference apt to be significant if small st. dev. of diff. bet. means and large sample sizes.
1	3.1	9.61	1.5	2.25	
2	3.7	13.69	1.6	2.56	
3	3.6	12.96	2.2	4.84	
4	2.7	7.29	1.7	2.89	
5	2.9	8.41	2.0	4	
6	3.0	9	1.8	3.24	
7	2.3	5.29	2.1	4.41	
8	2.6	6.76	1.6	2.56	
9	2.8	7.84	1.9	3.61	
10	3.0	9	2.1	4.41	
11	2.5	6.25	2.2	4.84	
12	2.9	8.41	1.4	1.96	
13	2.3	5.29	1.6	2.56	
14	2.8	7.84	1.7	2.89	
15	2.4	5.76	1.5	2.25	
16	2.6	6.76	1.6	2.56	
17	2.8	7.84	2.0	4	
18	3.3	10.89	2.1	4.41	
19	3.2	10.24	1.9	3.61	
20	3.3	10.89	2.0	4	

Size of sample n		20		20	Need NOT be same
Sum $X_i = \Sigma x_i = \Sigma x$		57.8		36.5	Sum of x's
Sample means $(\Sigma x_i)/n = \bar{x}$		2.89		1.825	The difference between these means will be the numerator of t ratio. (Absolute value.)
Sum of Squares $\Sigma(X_i)^2 = \Sigma x^2$		170.02		67.85	Sums of Squares
Square of sum $(\Sigma X_i)^2 = (\Sigma x)^2$		3340.8		1332.25	Squares of sums
$\dfrac{(\Sigma x)^2}{n}$		167.04		66.6125	"Grand mean" Also used in ANOVA
Σd^2		2.978		1.2375	$\Sigma d^2 = \Sigma x^2 - \dfrac{(\Sigma x)^2}{n}$ "SS$_T$"
Variances σ_1^2 and σ_2^2	Note one variance for EACH MEAN	0.1567		0.06513	$\sigma^2 = \Sigma d^2 / (n-1) =$ Variance.
σ_d^2		0.0111			$\sigma_d^2 = \dfrac{\sigma_1^2}{n_1} + \dfrac{\sigma_2^2}{n_2}$ "Pooled" variance of difference between
σ_d	Note ONE standard deviation.	0.1053			Square root of variance σ_d^2. Standard deviation of difference between means. Denominator.
$t_{computed}$		10.112	Ignore sign if negative. (Absolute value.)		$t = \dfrac{\bar{X}_1 - \bar{X}_2}{\sigma_d}$ The t ratio. Computed t.
df		19		19	Degrees of freedom. Each df = n - 1.

We have total of 38 degrees of freedom all together.

Table t for p=0.05 & 0.01 = 1.686 & 2.429. Since computed t is larger, **reject null hypothesis.**

Discussion

Though the full details of the applicable neuro-anatomy and physiology are not essential to this study, we note that the process behind this instance of Hering's law is very intricate. In terms of function, ostensibly the human visual system "abhors" a defocused image. In anthropomorphic terms, this effect translates into a corrective "effort," sufficiently potent to induce excess miosis and excess accommodation (as well as excess convergence, though not examined here). The brain "persistently seeks clear vision," and we can surmise that this process had evolutionary value.

In terms of anatomy, the visual system extends from the retina to the occipital cortex for its sensory component, and it involves various CNS nuclei, interconnections, and nerves for its motor part. [8, 9] Considering the retina to be the basic pertinent sensory structure, we know that nerve fibers branch off from the optic tracts and extend through the brachia of the superior colliculi to the pretectal nuclei. [10] Practitioners of neuro-ophthalmology already know that lesions posterior to ("downstream from") this branching do not disturb the pupillary reflex but affect vision, whereas lesions near and in the superior colliculi cause afferent pupillary dysfunctions without creating vision losses.

A pertinent anatomical detail is that both pretectal nuclei receive impulses from both retinae, and each pretectal nucleus initiates impulses to both Edinger-Westphal nuclei. That is to say, the neuronal connections are bilateral. Hence, for example, illuminating one eye constricts both pupils.

Meanwhile, the intra-orbital components of interest in this study, namely the pupils, the ciliary bodies and the medial rectus muscles, are all innervated by the oculomotor (third) cranial nerves that originate as a pair of oculomotor nuclei in the midbrain at the level of the superior colliculi.

These nerves emerge from their respective nuclei as two branches. Each superior branch eventually innervates the extraocular superior rectus muscle and the levator palperbrae muscle, so that it is not pertinent here.

The (larger) inferior branches have two neurofunctional components, somatic motor nerve fibers that end in the striated extraocular muscles including the medial recti, and pregangionic parasympathetic nerve fibers that end in the ciliary bodies, where there are synapses to postganglionic fibers in the ciliary body.

The pregangionic fibers originate in a specialized part of each oculomotor nucleus, the Edinger-Westphal nucleus, so that this nucleus supplies impulses bound for the pupil and the ciliary muscles. Pupillary miosis and accommodation appear to ensue from impulses that follow this route to the pupillary sphincter and ciliary muscle of each eye.

Sympathtic inneration is also obvious in the function of the pupil, specifically dilatation. Postganglionic fibers join the oculomotor nerve from the sympathetic plexus surrounding the internal carotid artery in the wall of the cavernous sinus.

In order to explain how Hering's law—at least as revealed in this study—links the size of the pupil with the accommodative state of that eye, we need only invoke the aforementioned afferent crisscross connections from the retinae to the Edinger-Westphal nuclei. Moreover, it is possible that there exist connections in the latter the between the fibers bound for the pupillary sphincters and those to the ciliary muscles. The point is that anatomy exists which can allow an excess effort for accommodation to cause excess miosis and excess effort for pupillary constriction to cause excess accommodation as found in this study.

Indeed, once sufficiently sensitive equipment was used, the results of this study were not elusive. Attempts 44 years ago with simpler equipment proved less successful, mainly because ideal measurements of the pupillary responses entail fractions of a millimeter. [2]

The argument can be made that the method of patient selection for this study favored the outcome obtained or at least exaggerated the results. This is a cogent point, but the goal was merely to demonstrate the applicability of Hering's law, even if merely under ideal conditions. Apparently factors such as age and fatigue do affect the near response, [11,8] but even without additional appropriate research and statistics it seems unreasonable to posit that the current results represent a physiologic aberration or an exception.

(Familiar ophthalmologic evidence for Hering's law arises in cases of strabismus in the form of the difference between primary and secondary deviations. [12] In that setting, Hering's law underpins a clinically useful diagnostic maneuver, but it affects only the extraocular muscles.)

Although all measurements without medication showed a high degree of right-left eye symmetry in these subjects, analysis of both miosis and accommodation under experimental conditions showed right-left discrepancies (evident, for example, in the OD vs. OS p-values). Presumably this incidental finding stems from eye dominance—all subjects were right-eye dominant—and in no case did it alter the principal outcomes or their statistical significance. In addition, care had been taken to randomize which eye was studied first.

Conclusion

Hering's law operates in the pupillary and accommodative components of the near reflex in healthy human subjects. Dilatation or cycloplegia of one eye fixating at near instigates significant excess miosis or excess accommodation in the other eye, as is predicted by the apparent physiologic mechanism behind Hering's law, and as is consistent with the neuro-anatomy of this part of the human visual system.

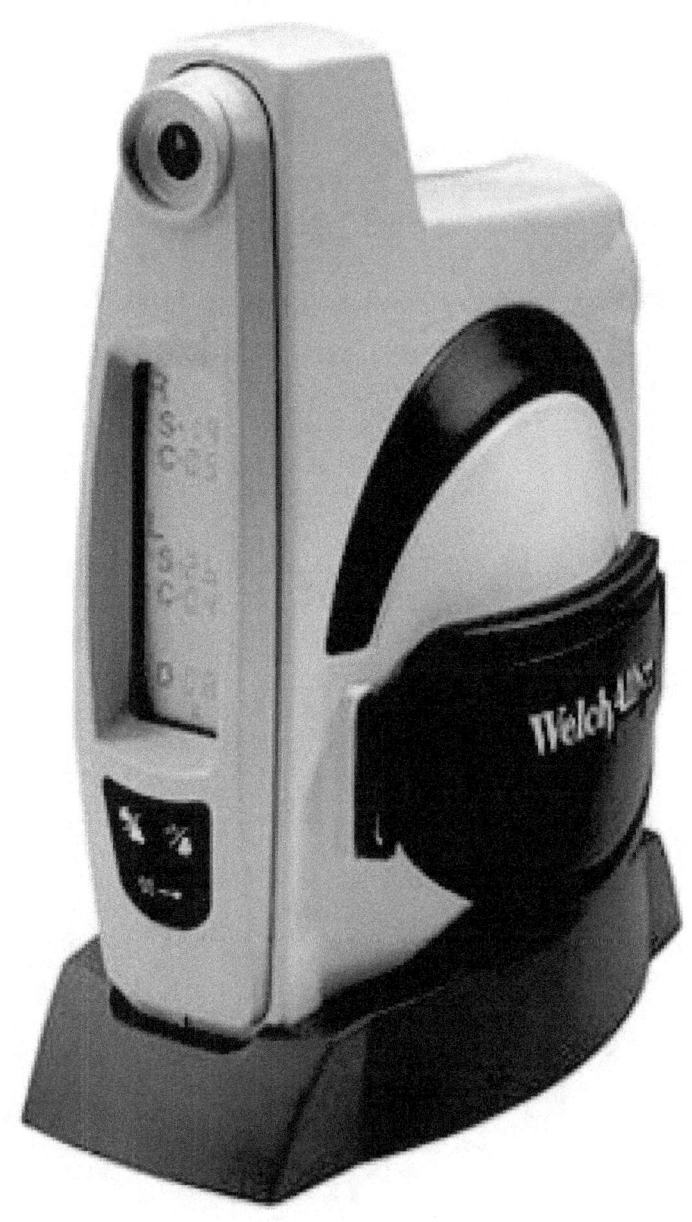

Welch-Allyn Autorefractor

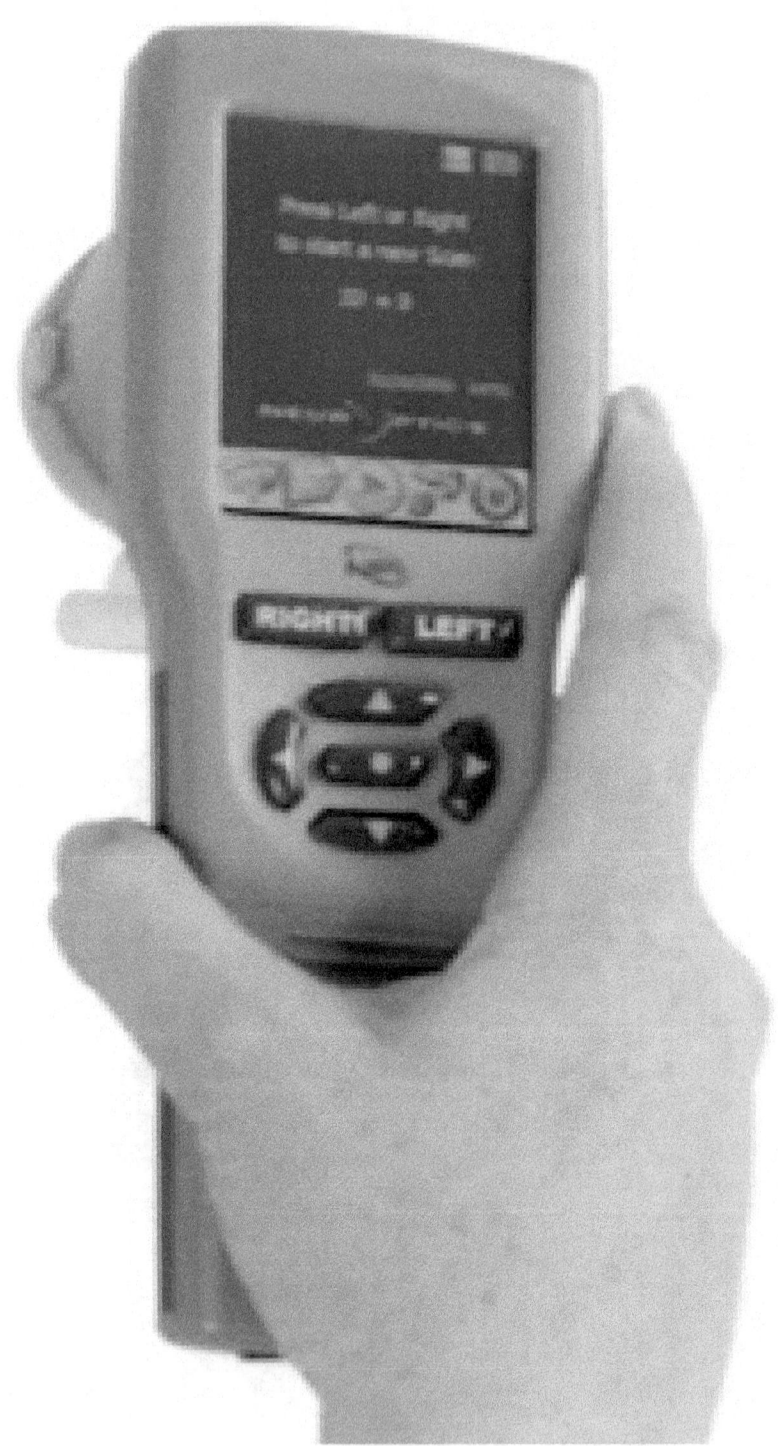

NeurOptics Pupillometer

Works Cited

---

[1] Cogan DG. Neurology of the ocular muscles. Springfield, Illinois: Charles C Thomas,

[2] Jagerman LS. Hering's law applied to the near reflex. *Am J Ophthalmol* 1970;70(4): 579-82.

[3] Schimitzek T, Wesemann W. Clinical evaluation of refraction using a handgeld wavefront autorefractor in young and adult patients. *Journal of Cataract and Refractive Surgery* 2002;28(9):1655-66. [The refractor under study was the SureSight device.]

[4] Walsh D, Block S, Rosanova L, Steele G, Ireland D. Comparison of the Welch Allyn SureSight to the Nikon Retinomax. *Optometry & Visual Science* 2001;78(12):83.

[5] Schallenberg M, Bangre V, Steuhl KP, Kremmer S, Selbach, JM. Comparison of the Colvard, Procyon and Neuroptics Pupillomoters for measuring pupil diameter under low ambient illumination. *J. Refactive Surgery* 2010;26(2):134-43.

[6] Saito S, Sotoyama M, Saitp S, Taptagaporn S. Physiologic indices of visual fatigue due to VDT operation: Pupillary reflexes and accommodative responses. *Industrial Health* 1994;32:57-66.

[7] Kasthurirangan S, Glasser A. Characteristic of the pupil responses during far-to-near and near-to-far accommodation. *Ophthalmic Physiol Opt* 2005;25(4):328-39.

[8] Fix JD. Neuroanatomy 4th ed. New York: Lippincott Williams & Wilkins, 2007:224-232.

[9] Richter HO, Costello P, Sponheim SR, Lee J, Pardo JV. Functional neuroanatomy of the human near/far response to blur cues. *Eur J. Neuroscience* 2004;20(10):2722-32.

[10] Martin, H. John. Neuroanatomy Text and Atlas. New York McGraw Hill, 2012: Sections on Oculomotor Nerve.

[11] Wilhelm H, Schaeffel F, Wilhelm B. Age dependence of the pupillary near reflex. *Klin Monbl Augenheilkunde* 1993;203(2):110-6.

[12] Wright KW, Spiegel PH. Pediatric ophthalmology and strabismus. Second edition. New York: Springer Verlag, 2003:191.

Please note that an internet search readily provides diagrams and pictures of the pertinent brain and orbital anatomy, in addition to the works listed above.

Reprints of my original (1970) paper are no longer available.

www.ingramcontent.com/pod-product-compliance
Lightning Source LLC
Chambersburg PA
CBHW080630180526
45168CB00007B/3107